Osteopathy Treatment

Treating Back, Knee and Chronic Pain Using Osteopathic Spinal Manipulation Techniques

Dan Phillips PhD

~LARRY~

For your unwavering support, encouragement, and friendship. Your presence in my life has been a constant source of inspiration. Thank you for your invaluable kindness and belief in my journey. This book is a token of appreciation for your enduring friendship and steadfast encouragement.

TABLE OF CONTENT

° Detailed Description of Osteopathic Spinal Manipulation Techniques for Addressing Various Types of Back Pain

° Illustrative Case Examples Showcasing the Application of Techniques for Specific Back Pain Etiologies

° Consideration of Patient Safety and Contraindications in Performing Spinal Manipulations

°°Part V: Osteopathic Management of Knee Pain: Techniques and Protocols°°

5. Osteopathic Management of Knee Pain: Techniques and Protocols

° Exploration of Osteopathic Techniques Aimed at Alleviating Knee Pain and Improving Joint Function

° Discussion of Manual Methods to Address Common Knee Conditions

° Integration of Osteopathic Treatment with Rehabilitative Exercises for Comprehensive Knee Pain Management

CHAPTER 1

Introduction to Osteopathic Spinal Manipulation Techniques

With its roots in a long tradition of holistic medicine, osteopathic medicine provides a distinctive method of treating patients that stresses the body's innate ability to heal itself and the interconnection of all of its systems. Osteopathic spine manipulation is the cornerstone method that is at the heart of this approach. It has the potential to improve overall well-being, reduce pain, and restore mobility. This chapter explores the history, tenets, and possible uses of osteopathic spinal manipulation, laying the groundwork for a thorough examination of how it might be used to treat chronic pain in the knees, back, and other body parts.

Short Overview of Osteopathy's History: Holistic Underpinnings

Dr. Andrew Taylor Still established osteopathy in the late 19th century in reaction to the shortcomings of the time's accepted medical methods. The goal of Dr. Still's groundbreaking viewpoint was to see the body as a single unit in which the interaction of its anatomical, functional, and circulatory components was crucial to both health and illness. Osteopathy adopted a holistic perspective, acknowledging the body's inherent capacity for self-regulation and healing, and rejected reductionist methods. The osteopathic spinal manipulation, a manual method intended to support the body's inherent healing mechanisms, was made possible by this historical basis.

Basic Ideas of Osteopathic Spinal Manipulation

Fundamental principles form the basis of osteopathic spinal manipulation and serve as guidelines for its practice. The first premise is the idea of the body's self-regulation system, in which structural and functional abnormalities can result in deteriorated health. Osteopathic physicians feel that by giving the spine its natural alignment and mobility back, the body's self-healing powers can be triggered, aiding in healing and relieving pain.

The second concept highlights the connection between the anatomy and physiology of the organism. Based on the knowledge that physical disruptions, such as misalignments or limitations in spinal segments, can exacerbate pain and dysfunction, osteopathic spine manipulation was developed. Osteopaths use precise techniques to gently manipulate these segments in an effort to restore normal biomechanics and optimal bodily function.

The idea of the body's fluid dynamics is at the heart of the third principle. The goal of osteopathic spinal manipulation is to improve lymphatic and circulatory flow, which will facilitate the elimination of waste and the supply of nutrients. This method aids in both tissue repair and inflammation reduction, which is a common cause of pain.

The advantages and possible consequences of osteopathic spinal manipulation

For those who are in pain, osteopathic spinal manipulation has several potential advantages, especially when it comes to chronic pain in the knee, back, and other areas. Pain relief and increased joint mobility can be achieved with this therapy by correcting structural imbalances and constraints. Furthermore, because osteopathic medicine is holistic in nature, practitioners take into account a patient's entire health environment, which includes lifestyle choices, mental health, and psychosocial effects.

Osteopathic spinal manipulation has been shown to have the potential to release endorphins, which are the body's natural analgesics, so providing instantaneous pain relief. Moreover, manipulation's increased circulation can aid in tissue repair and lessen the accumulation of inflammatory chemicals, which will help with long-term pain management.

Osteopathic medicine frequently includes patient empowerment and education in addition to medical benefits. In order to maintain optimal spinal health, patients are advised to actively participate in their recovery process and embrace methods including ergonomic habits, exercise, and stress management.

Osteopathic spine manipulation has the potential to lessen the need for invasive surgeries or pharmaceutical interventions in the field of pain management. In line with patients' preferences for all-natural, non-invasive remedies, osteopathic treatment provides a holistic alternative by addressing the root causes of pain and reestablishing bodily equilibrium.

The first chapter concludes by laying the groundwork for a thorough examination of osteopathic spinal manipulation methods for the management of chronic pain in the knees, back, and other body parts. Osteopathy, with its foundation in a holistic philosophy and guiding principles, is a distinct pain treatment method that seeks to reestablish the body's natural ability to heal. For those looking for comprehensive and efficient ways to address their pain, osteopathic spinal manipulation is a viable option because of its capacity to reduce pain, increase mobility, and boost general well-being.

CHAPTER 2

Understanding Back, Knee, and Chronic Pain: A Comprehensive Overview

A person's quality of life can be significantly impacted by pain, which is a common human experience resulting from a complex interplay of physiological, psychological, and environmental elements. Pain from the musculoskeletal system, especially in the back and knee areas, is one of the most common and incapacitating kinds of pain. In order to provide readers a thorough grasp of the underlying causes, contributing variables, and complex interactions between biomechanics, posture, and pain, Chapter 2 of this book explores the complex realm of back, knee, and chronic pain.

Peeling Back the Layers: Causes and Contributing Factors of Pain

Examining the various sources of pain is the first step towards understanding its origins. Even while pain frequently appears to be localized, it usually stems from a complex network of interrelated variables. In the development of musculoskeletal pain, a number of factors are important, including genetics, lifestyle, work, trauma, and medical history.

For example, genetic predisposition can affect the structure of ligaments, joints, and bones, rendering some people more prone to particular kinds of pain. Lifestyle decisions including insufficient exercise, bad diet, and sedentary behavior might make this vulnerability worse. These variables raise the chance of obesity, which in turn raises the risk of musculoskeletal pain, especially in the knee and back areas.

Occupational aspects are also important to consider. Prolonged sitting, repeated motions, or heavy lifting are among the jobs that can cause strain on the knee and back joints, which over time can result in chronic discomfort. Similar to this, trauma from events like sports injuries or accidents can cause pain that develops right away or later on and lasts for a long time.

Common Painful Conditions and Musculoskeletal Disorders

In the field of musculoskeletal pain, a multitude of diseases and ailments are prominent. In-depth discussion of these ailments' causes and physiological effects is provided in Chapter 2.

To start with the back, lumbar disc herniation is one of the most common conditions. This happens when the discs that act as cushions between the vertebrae burst or bulge, applying pressure on the surrounding nerves and producing localized pain. Degenerative disc disease is another common culprit, where chronic discomfort and decreased mobility are caused by the discs in the spine naturally wearing down. The irregular curvature of the spine known as scoliosis can cause back discomfort because the vertebrae are not aligned properly.

On the other hand, osteoarthritis, a degenerative joint condition that erodes the cartilage cushioning the knee joints, is frequently associated with knee pain. When there is bone-on-bone contact as a result of this erosion, severe discomfort and limited mobility result. Often referred to as "runner's knee," patellofemoral pain syndrome is a condition that can affect both athletes and non-athletes due to abnormal kneecap placement. Severe knee discomfort and instability can be brought on by ligament injuries, such as tears to the anterior cruciate ligament (ACL).

Persistent pain, whether it comes from the knee or the back, adds another level of difficulty. It frequently arises from a complex interaction between neurological, emotional, and physical variables. Over time, the nervous system may become sensitized, intensifying pain signals and starting a vicious cycle of ongoing suffering.

Posture, Biomechanics, and the Dancing of Pain

An essential connection between pain and the body's mechanics is made via posture and biomechanics. Understanding the interactions between these components is crucial to figuring out the cause of musculoskeletal pain, as chapter 2 demonstrates.

The study of biomechanics, or how the body's structures move and work, can help explain the causes of pain. Muscle imbalances, incorrect movement patterns, and poor posture can all interfere with the body's natural mechanics and put stress on the muscles, ligaments, and joints. For example, extended use of smartphones and desk work can cause forward head posture, which can strain the muscles in the neck and upper back and cause chronic pain.

More than merely a matter of alignment, posture is a dynamic representation of our emotional and psychological well-being. Anxiety, despair, and stress can all lead to bad posture, which can worsen discomfort. When emotional stress materializes as physical tightness, creating a vicious cycle of tension and suffering, the mind-body connection is evident.

Finitude

Readers can find a thorough examination of the intricacies related to chronic pain, knee pain, and back pain in Chapter 2. It reveals the complex network of variables that lead to these kinds of pain, ranging from traumatic events and job demands to heredity and lifestyle decisions. The chapter highlights the range of illnesses that can result in severe pain by exploring the field of common musculoskeletal ailments. It also highlights the critical role that posture and biomechanics play, showing how these factors interact to influence how people experience pain.

Understanding the complex nature of pain helps people become more aware of their bodies and possible causes of their misery. Equipped with this understanding, readers can set out on a path of management, prevention, and even change. Through educated decisions about exercise, lifestyle, and mental health, the complex dance of pain can be guided toward alleviation and healing.

CHAPTER 3

Assessment and Diagnosis of Pain Conditions: A Osteopathic Approach

- Step-by-step guide to conducting a thorough osteopathic assessment for pain conditions.

- Integration of patient history, physical examination, and diagnostic imaging in determining the root cause of pain.

- **Differentiation between acute and chronic pain presentations for tailored treatment approaches.**

Since pain is a complicated and subjective sensation with many underlying causes, a precise diagnosis and assessment are essential to the development of a successful treatment plan. In the field of osteopathic medicine, a thorough evaluation of pain is critical. In order to identify the underlying causes of pain, this chapter explores the complexities of doing an extensive osteopathic assessment for pain disorders. It emphasizes the integration of diagnostic imaging, physical examination, and patient history. It also discusses how important it is to differentiate between acute and chronic pain presentations in order to develop individualized treatment plans.

A Comprehensive Guide to the Osteopathic Assessment Process

The knowledge that pain is frequently an indication of structural abnormalities, limitations, or dysfunctions inside the body is fundamental to the osteopathic method. To find these fundamental problems, a methodical assessment procedure is used. The first step in the assessment is a thorough review of the patient's medical history, during which the professional will ascertain the type, location, duration, and start of the pain. This story may disclose triggers or predisposing variables in addition to providing context for the pain.

The patient's narrative is followed by a thorough physical examination. Numerous tests are included in this examination, such as neurological evaluation, range of motion testing, postural analysis, and probing of soft tissues and bone landmarks. Osteopathic physicians can uncover regions of malfunction or asymmetry in the body and obtain important insights into the causes that contribute to pain by methodically assessing the body's biomechanics.

Combining Laboratory and Diagnostic Imaging

To further understand the underlying cause of pain, laboratory testing or diagnostic imaging may occasionally be recommended by the osteopathic examination. The diagnosis of structural anomalies, joint deterioration, or disc herniation can be facilitated by the precise view of anatomical structures provided by imaging modalities like X-rays, MRIs, or ultrasounds. On the other hand, laboratory testing may be used to evaluate inflammatory markers that may be linked to pain or to rule out systemic illnesses.

It is crucial to remember that, even if laboratory and diagnostic imaging procedures can yield insightful data, their best results come from a combination with a clinical evaluation. Osteopathy promotes a comprehensive understanding of pain that takes into account both structural and functional factors. As such, diagnostic test results should be evaluated in the context of this larger understanding.

Differing Between Presentations of Acute and Chronic Pain

Making the distinction between acute and chronic pain presentations is a crucial part of the osteopathic assessment process. Recent wounds, inflammations, or tissue damage are common causes of acute discomfort, which can also have a clear physiological foundation. The goals of osteopathic treatment for acute pain are to minimize discomfort, lower inflammation, and promote tissue repair via soft tissue techniques, gentle manipulation, and other methods.

On the other hand, chronic pain is defined by ongoing suffering that does not go away as quickly as one may think. Complex interplay between psychological, social, and physical elements are frequently involved. Osteopathic treatment of chronic pain necessitates a more all-encompassing strategy that takes into account the patient's emotional health, way of life, and coping methods in addition to the structural issues. Strategies for stress management, relaxation, and patient education may be used in conjunction with techniques targeted at regaining proper biomechanics, enhancing circulation, and modifying pain pathways.

In summary, an osteopathic perspective on pain management necessitates a thorough and comprehensive approach to examination and diagnosis. Osteopathic physicians can identify the underlying causes of pain by methodically integrating historical information from the patient, physical examination, and, if required, diagnostic imaging. Furthermore, being able to distinguish between acute and chronic pain presentations enables the development of specialized treatment plans that address pain's larger psychosocial and emotional components in addition to its physical manifestations. This all-encompassing method lays the groundwork for efficient and patient-focused pain management within the osteopathic field.

CHAPTER 4

Osteopathic Spinal Manipulation Techniques for Back Pain

- Detailed description of osteopathic spinal manipulation techniques for addressing various types of back pain.

- Illustrative case examples showcasing the application of techniques for specific back pain etiologies.

- **Consideration of patient safety and contraindications in performing spinal manipulations.**

A common and frequently incapacitating ailment that affects millions of people globally is back pain. Although there are many different ways to treat back pain, osteopathic spinal manipulation techniques have become well-known for their ability to effectively relieve the condition. This chapter explores the nuances of these methods, providing a thorough analysis of their use, real-world examples, and the critical issue of patient safety.

The Osteopathic Spinal Manipulation Art and Science

The osteopathic theory that the body has an inherent capacity for self-healing is the foundation of osteopathic spinal manipulation treatments. With the hands-on technique, balance is restored, pain is decreased, and general well-being is improved by expert physical manipulation of the spine and surrounding tissues. The methods focus on the musculoskeletal system with the goals of enhancing nervous system performance, releasing muscular tension, and enhancing joint mobility.

Methods for Various Kinds of Back Pain

The first section of the chapter explores a variety of osteopathic spine manipulation procedures, each designed to treat a particular kind of back pain.

1. Direct Thrust Technique: Also referred to as high-velocity, low-amplitude thrust (HVLA), this technique involves applying a swift, controlled force to a particular joint in order to realign it properly. It is frequently used to treat acute back pain brought on by muscle spasms or joint misalignments.

2. The Muscle Energy Technique: This method requires the patient's full engagement. To relieve tension

and regain joint mobility, the patient contracts a particular muscle while the practitioner delivers counterforce. It is very helpful for joint limitations and muscular imbalances.

3. Myofascial Release: This method works on the fascia, a connective tissue that can get stressed out or injured over time, causing it to tighten and constrict. The practitioner's goal is to release fascia tension through the application of gentle, sustained pressure, which will reduce pain and restore flexibility.

Example Cases: Using Methods for Particular Back Pain Etiologies

Techniques outlined are given a practical dimension through illustrative case studies. Take the case of a patient who has severe lower back pain as a result of a misaligned lumbar joint. One possible method is the direct thrust approach, in which the physician applies a precise force to realign the injured joint. Readers are given insight into the possible consequences and the methodical process of applying techniques through this case study.

In a different situation, the muscle energy approach might be helpful for a patient who has chronic upper back discomfort brought on by muscular imbalances. In order to increase joint mobility and reduce discomfort, the practitioner gently applies resistance while guiding the patient in tightening particular muscles. These case studies highlight the adaptability of osteopathic spinal manipulation methods and their capacity to treat a wide range of back pain causes.

Discontinuities and Patient Safety

Although there may be advantages to osteopathic spinal manipulation procedures, patient safety comes first. In-depth information about precautions and contraindications that practitioners should take into account before using these procedures is covered in this chapter. To maintain patient well-being, conditions like osteoporosis, recent fractures, and certain neurological illnesses call for careful assessment and technique adaption.

The chapter also emphasizes how important having the right education and experience is. Osteopathic practitioners get extensive study and training in order to acquire the skills required for applying these procedures in a safe and efficient manner. It is important to remind readers that only licensed medical experts who are capable of appropriately assessing a patient's condition and customizing treatments should undertake spinal manipulation.

Finitude

In Chapter 4, osteopathic spinal manipulation techniques are explored as a useful tool for treating different kinds of back pain. Through thorough technique descriptions, insightful case studies, and a focus on patient safety concerns, the chapter provides readers with a thorough comprehension of this methodology. As osteopathic spinal manipulators and their patients travel the road toward pain alleviation, increased mobility, and greater well-being, the art and science of the technique come to life.

CHAPTER 5

Osteopathic Management of
Knee Pain: Techniques and
Protocols

- Exploration of osteopathic techniques aimed at alleviating knee pain and improving joint function.

- Discussion of manual methods to address common knee conditions, such as osteoarthritis,

ligament injuries, and meniscal tears.

- Integration of osteopathic treatment with rehabilitative exercises for comprehensive knee pain management.

The knees are complex weight-bearing joints that are essential to the body's overall functionality and movement. They are, nevertheless, vulnerable to a number of ailments that may cause them discomfort or damage. Osteopathic medicine provides a comprehensive approach to treating knee pain, including a variety of methods intended to reduce pain, strengthen joints, and improve quality of life in general. The many osteopathic approaches used to treat knee pain are examined in this chapter, along with manual techniques that target common knee disorders. The integration of osteopathic treatment with rehabilitative exercises is emphasized as a means of providing comprehensive knee pain management.

An Examination of Osteopathic Knee Pain Management

An extensive examination is the first step in the osteopathic treatment of knee pain in order to determine the underlying sources of discomfort. Various osteopathic treatments can be used to address the specific problems causing knee discomfort once the underlying reasons have been identified. These therapies, which work to improve joint mobility, lessen muscle tension, and restore appropriate alignment, frequently include manual manipulation, soft tissue mobilization, and other hands-on procedures.

Joint mobilization, which entails very mild and controlled movements of the knee joint, is one often employed approach. Osteopathic physicians can assist restore normal joint mechanics, lessen stiffness, and increase range of motion by using precise pressures. To treat muscle imbalances and relieve stress in the knee area, soft tissue methods like trigger point therapy and myofascial release are also employed.

Manual Techniques for Typical Knee Issues

Osteopathic medicine offers a focused method for treating particular knee issues that frequently result in pain. Degenerative joint diseases like osteoarthritis can cause discomfort, inflammation, and decreased joint function. The goals of osteopathic treatment are to enhance the surrounding muscle support, decrease inflammation, and improve joint biomechanics. Myofascial release and joint mobilization are two methods that can be used to improve knee function and reduce discomfort.

ACL rips are one type of ligament injury that can be brought on by traumatizing incidents or engaging in sports. Osteopathic treatment include a thorough evaluation of the biomechanics and stability of the ligaments, followed by methods designed to accelerate healing and restore stability. Rehabilitative exercises and manual techniques can be used in tandem to progressively strengthen the damaged ligament and surrounding muscles.

Another common knee problem is meniscal tears, which can cause pain, swelling, and mechanical symptoms. Gentle manipulation is used in osteopathic treatment to correct joint alignment and reduce meniscus stress. Soft tissue approaches can also improve blood flow and lessen muscle guarding to aid in the healing process.

Combining Rehabilitation and Osteopathic Treatment

Comprehensive knee pain care includes both preventing future problems and restoring optimal function in addition to treating current discomfort. To accomplish these ends, osteopathic treatment combines well with rehabilitative exercises. The main goals of rehabilitation programs are to increase joint stability, improve mobility generally, and strengthen the muscles surrounding the knee.

Osteopathic physicians collaborate extensively with their patients to create customized workout regimens that enhance the manual therapy methods administered in-person. Proprioceptive training, range-of-motion exercises, strengthening exercises, and functional motions that imitate everyday activities are a few examples of these exercises. Osteopathic medicine and rehabilitation work together to provide patients with a comprehensive care plan that not only reduces pain but also gives them the tools they need to take an active role in their own healing.

To sum up, osteopathic treatment of knee pain represents a thorough strategy that includes a range of methods and procedures. Osteopathic physicians provide manual treatment for common knee disorders include meniscal tears, osteoarthritis, and ligament injuries with the goal of reducing discomfort and enhancing joint function. Furthermore, a comprehensive and patient-centered approach to knee pain management is ensured by the combination of osteopathic treatment and rehabilitation exercises. By using this all-encompassing method, people with knee pain can improve their mobility and general well-being in addition to receiving pain relief.

CHAPTER 6

Chronic Pain Management through Osteopathic Care

- Comprehensive approach to managing chronic pain using osteopathic principles and techniques.

- Examination of the role of osteopathy in addressing pain sensitization, central nervous system changes, and psychosocial factors.

- Incorporation of patient education and self-care strategies to promote long-term pain relief.

The illness known as chronic pain is widespread and intricate, and it can significantly affect a person's quality of life. For the treatment of chronic pain, osteopathic care offers a thorough and all-encompassing approach, whereas conventional methods frequently concentrate on symptom suppression. In order to treat the complex nature of chronic pain, this chapter explores the integration of osteopathic principles and procedures. This chapter looks at issues ranging from pain sensitization to psychosocial variables and how osteopathic treatment can help people feel better and take back control of their life.

A Comprehensive Method for Treating Persistent Pain

The idea that the body is an interconnected system and that problems in one area can have an impact on other areas is one that osteopathic medicine embraces. This holistic approach has a clear benefit when it comes to managing chronic pain. Osteopathy aims to locate and treat the underlying causes of pain rather than only treating its symptoms in order to provide long-term relief.

Pain Sensitization and Modifications to the Central Nervous System

Complex neurobiological changes, such as pain sensitization and modifications in the central nervous system's pain signal processing, are frequently associated with chronic pain. Osteopathic medicine acknowledges these occurrences and uses methods to bring back normal sensory function. By restoring neuronal connections to their normal state, mild manual adjustments can lower pain amplification and raise pain threshold.

Psychosocial Aspects: The Mind-Body Link in Pain Treatment

The foundation of osteopathic medicine is the complex link between mental and physical health. This chapter explores the psychosocial aspects of chronic pain, including the role that emotional stressors, despair, and anxiety may have in the persistence of pain. Osteopathic physicians are educated to evaluate a patient's mental condition in addition to their physical symptoms since they understand that treating psychosocial issues might improve pain management.

Including Self-Care Techniques and Patient Education

The foundation of osteopathic treatment for chronic pain management is empowerment. Patients are better able to take an active role in their own recovery when they are informed about their disease, the causes of their pain, and self-care techniques. Patients are coached in self-care practices that supplement the hands-on treatments delivered by osteopathic practitioners. These practices range from ergonomic adjustments and posture awareness to stress management strategies and gentle exercises.

Sample Cases: Getting Around in the World of Chronic Pain

The chapter provides case studies of individuals with various chronic pain problems to demonstrate how osteopathic care can be applied to chronic pain management. These illustrations explain how osteopathic methods, such as myofascial release and cranial manipulations, can be combined to treat psychological issues that lead to pain persistence in addition to physical discomfort. Readers are able to understand the subtle methods necessary to customize osteopathic treatment to each patient's demands by looking at these cases.

A Way to Get Pain Relief That Lasts

The collaborative nature of managing chronic pain with osteopathic care is highlighted in the chapter's conclusion. It emphasizes the value of collaborations between patients and practitioners, in which the course of treatment is determined by mutual understanding and common objectives. Osteopathy provides a framework for navigating the complicated terrain of chronic pain by seeing pain as a multifaceted experience that has the capacity to bring about both radical healing and pain alleviation. As patients adopt self-care techniques and professionals assist them in regaining equilibrium, the pursuit of long-term pain alleviation transforms into an empowered and comprehensive undertaking.

CHAPTER 7

Special Considerations and

Patient Populations

- Exploration of osteopathic treatment considerations for specific patient populations, such as pediatric, geriatric, and pregnant individuals.

- Discussion of adapting techniques for patients with comorbidities and unique challenges.

- **Ethical considerations in treating pain-related conditions within the osteopathic scope of practice.**

Osteopathic medicine applies its ideas to a wide spectrum of patient populations because of its focus on personalized treatment plans and holistic care. This chapter explores the complex realm of osteopathic treatment considerations for particular populations, such as children, the elderly, and expectant mothers. It addresses the ethical issues that support pain-related therapy within the osteopathic scope of practice and examines the art of tailoring approaches for patients with comorbidities and particular obstacles.

Entire Lifetime Osteopathic Assistance

Pregnant, elderly, and pediatric patients have distinct physiological and biomechanical needs that call for customized osteopathic treatment methods. Young patients need to be treated with age- and gentleness-appropriate methods that honor their growing musculoskeletal systems. Children's osteopathic treatment seeks to promote healthy growth and development while addressing common problems such musculoskeletal discomfort, postural abnormalities, and sports injuries.

Conversely, age-related ailments and degenerative changes are frequently faced by geriatric individuals. Osteopathic physicians customize their treatment plans to increase range of motion, reduce discomfort, and promote joint health. Strategies could center on preserving functional autonomy, averting falls, and alleviating discomforts associated with aging.

Pregnant people undergo particular musculoskeletal alterations as well as postural adjustments. Promoting pelvic alignment, reducing stress on supporting ligaments, and treating discomfort related to postural changes are the main goals of osteopathic therapy during pregnancy. Methods are modified to protect and comfort the growing fetus as well as the expectant mother.

Tailoring Strategies to Comorbidities and Particular Difficulties

Osteopathic patients with comorbidities—diabetes, autoimmune diseases, or cardiovascular conditions—need a careful approach to treatment. Osteopathic physicians take into account how pain, illness, and therapy interact, adapting their methods to protect patients and avoid making underlying illnesses worse. To create integrated care plans that meet these people's complex demands, cooperation with other healthcare professionals becomes crucial.

A patient-centered approach is necessary to address special problems including cultural concerns, psychological factors, or cognitive disabilities. Osteopathic physicians are sensitive and flexible in how they adjust their methods to the unique needs of each patient. A more thorough and fruitful treatment experience is facilitated by effective communication and a detailed comprehension of the patient's history.

Ethical Matters in Osteopathic Pain Therapy

Osteopathic medicine is governed by a set of moral precepts that place an emphasis on patient autonomy, welfare, and the obligation of the practitioner to deliver high-quality care. In the context of pain management, informed consent, patient education, and collaborative decision-making are all important ethical factors to take into account. Osteopathic doctors have candid conversations with their patients to make sure they are aware of the possible advantages, disadvantages, and available treatment options.

Moreover, the management of pain with pharmaceutical interventions and referrals is also subject to ethical problems. Following professional rules and legal requirements, osteopathic practitioners work in conjunction with patients to select the most appropriate and effective course of action.

The chapter on patient groups and unique considerations concludes by highlighting how flexible osteopathic care is. Osteopathic practitioners offer patient-centered and comprehensive care by investigating the special needs of young patients, the elderly, and expectant mothers. They also customize their procedures for patients with comorbidities and special difficulties. Steeped in moral values, osteopathic pain treatment works to enhance people's health from a variety of backgrounds and stages of life while developing a strong therapeutic alliance based on empathy, healing, and trust.

CHAPTER 8

Evidence-Based Practice and Future Directions in Osteopathic Pain Management

- **Examination of current research and clinical evidence supporting the efficacy of osteopathic spinal manipulation for pain relief.**

- **Integration of emerging technologies and advancements**

in pain management within the osteopathic framework.

- Reflection on the potential evolution of osteopathic techniques and their role in interdisciplinary pain management approaches.

The role of osteopathic care in promoting well-being and offering relief from pain is always changing in tandem with the field of pain management. The foundations of evidence-based treatment in osteopathic pain management are examined in this chapter, along with the state of research and clinical data that attest to the effectiveness of osteopathic spine manipulation. Additionally, it looks to the future of this field by taking into account the incorporation of cutting-edge technologies, the advancement of osteopathic methods, and their role in multidisciplinary approaches to pain management.

Research-Based Methodology: Adproving Osteopathic Pain Treatment

In a time where evidence-based practice is valued highly, it is essential to confirm the effectiveness of osteopathic pain management methods. The first part of the chapter reviews the literature and clinical trials that support the use of osteopathic spinal manipulation for a range of pain conditions, such as headaches, neck pain, and back pain. Osteopathic care can be included in pain management regimens because of the research this chapter presents on pain reduction, improved functional results, and patient satisfaction.

Welcoming Advances in Technology

As technology develops, there are exciting new opportunities for its integration within the osteopathic framework. Wearable technology, biofeedback systems, and virtual reality present fresh opportunities to improve patient participation and treatment results. Virtual reality settings, for example, can help patients unwind during osteopathic treatments, and wearable technology could monitor movements and posture to help tailor treatment regimens. Osteopathic physicians can better customize their treatments and provide patients more control over how they manage their pain by utilizing these technology.

The History of Osteopathic Methods

Osteopathic methods are dynamic; they change and progress in response to new discoveries in science as well as shifting demands from patients. This chapter explores how osteopathic treatments may develop in the future and how knowledge from biomechanics and neuroscience may influence the development of practical therapies. Personalized therapy regimens that take into account a patient's genetic composition, lifestyle choices, and pain management mechanisms may result from the integration of precision medicine concepts. Osteopathic practitioners aim to obtain even more customized pain treatment outcomes by refining their procedures and welcoming new knowledge while being open to innovation.

Multidisciplinary Techniques for Pain Management

With the realization that no one method can fully address the complexity of chronic pain, the future of pain care is intrinsically multidisciplinary. With its emphasis on the whole person, osteopathic medicine is ideally suited for working in tandem with other medical specialties like physical therapy, psychotherapy, and integrative medicine. The chapter considers the possibilities of multidisciplinary approaches to pain management, in which osteopathic methods are an important part of an all-encompassing therapy regimen. Practitioners can address the multifaceted nature of pain and give patients a comprehensive toolkit for healing by collaborating with one another.

Recap: Shaping the Future of Pain Management

The development of osteopathic pain management is summarized in Chapter 8, from its evidence-based beginnings to its incorporation of cutting-edge technologies and interdisciplinary cooperation. Osteopathic physicians are shaping the future of pain management as they promote patient care through constant method improvement, technological adaptation, and teamwork. Osteopathic practitioners can negotiate the changing environment of pain care by staying rooted in the holistic concepts that drive their profession.

This allows them to provide patients with not only pain relief but also the possibility of transformative healing and enhanced quality of life.